ORGANIC DIET PLAN GUIDE BOOK

Improve Your Health and Transform Your Well-being with the Organic Diet

LARRY HERMAN

Table of Contents

Introduction

An "organic diet" is a dietary approach that prioritizes the consumption of organic foods. Organic farming include agricultural methods that refrain from utilizing synthetic pesticides, herbicides, genetically modified organisms (GMOs), and synthetic fertilizers. Organic farmers employ natural techniques such as crop rotation, composting, and biological pest management to sustain soil fertility and regulate pest populations.

Here are fundamental elements to comprehend regarding the organic diet:

• **Certification for organic products:** Numerous countries, such as the

United States, Europe, and others, have stringent restrictions that dictate the usage of the term "organic." In order to obtain organic certification, farms and food producers are required to comply with certain regulations. This certification guarantees that the food has been cultivated in accordance with organic agricultural regulations.

• The primary motivation for individuals opting for an organic diet is to minimize their contact with artificial pesticides and herbicides. Organic farming employs natural techniques to manage pests, such as the introduction of beneficial insects or the implementation of companion planting practices.

Organic foods are cultivated without the utilization of genetically modified organisms, making them GMO-free. Consequently, organic farming ensures that crops and animals have not undergone genetic modification to achieve particular characteristics, and the cultivation of genetically modified seeds is strictly forbidden.

• Soil health is prioritized in organic farming through strategies such as crop rotation, cover cropping, and the application of compost and organic materials. Optimal soil health enhances the overall nutritional value of the food that is cultivated.

• Organic meat, dairy, and eggs prioritize the ethical treatment of animals, focusing on their welfare. Organic standards often encompass criteria such as provision of outdoor access, adequate space, and limitations on the utilization of antibiotics and growth hormones.

• Organic farming endeavors to mitigate its environmental impact by refraining from the use of synthetic chemicals and advocating for sustainable practices. This encompasses the actions of decreasing water consumption, advocating for the preservation of diverse ecosystems, and mitigating the process of soil erosion.

• **Nutritional Content:** The question of whether organic foods are more healthy than conventionally cultivated foods is still being debated. However, some studies indicate that organic produce may contain higher amounts of specific nutrients and antioxidants.

It is crucial to emphasize that the organic label primarily emphasizes the production processes rather than the total nutritional value of the food. Incorporating an organic diet into a healthy lifestyle is beneficial, but it is crucial to also take into account one's overall dietary choices, which should include a diverse range of foods that are high in nutrients, regardless of whether they are organic or not. Furthermore, an individual's inclination towards organic products may be influenced by their own interests, values, and availability of such products.

CHAPTER ONE
Definition of Organic

The term "organic" can have multiple interpretations depending on the specific circumstances. Here are few typical applications of the term:

1. **Chemistry:** In the field of chemistry, the term "organic" is used to describe substances that consist of carbon atoms, which are usually obtained from living creatures. Organic chemistry is the field of chemistry that focuses on the study of molecules that include carbon.

2. **Agriculture:** In the field of agriculture, the term "organic" pertains to a farming technique that abstains from employing synthetic

pesticides, herbicides, fertilizers, and genetically modified organisms (GMOs). Organic farming, in contrast, utilizes natural techniques to foster soil well-being, manage pests, and improve long-term viability.

3. Food and Diet: In the realm of food and diet, the term "organic" typically pertains to food items that have been cultivated using organic farming methods. Organic foods are often devoid of artificial chemicals and genetically modified organisms (GMOs), and they can be officially certified as such by regulatory authorities.

4. General Usage: In common parlance, the term "organic" is occasionally employed in a broader sense to refer to anything that is natural, unaltered, or devoid of artificial additions. For instance, individuals may use the term "organic" while discussing skincare products or cleaning materials, expressing a preference for items that are believed to be more natural or environmentally conscious.

It is crucial to take into account the particular context in which the term "organic" is employed in order to ascertain its exact significance. The understanding of the term might vary, whether it pertains to chemistry, agriculture, food, or common usage.

Organic Certification

Organic certification is a process through which agricultural products, including crops and livestock, are verified as meeting specific organic standards. The certification assures consumers that the food or other agricultural products labeled as "organic" have been produced in accordance with established organic farming practices. These standards vary slightly between countries and regions, but they generally share common principles.

Here is a general overview of the organic certification process:

Adherence to Standards:

• Farmers and food producers must adhere to specific organic farming standards outlined by regulatory bodies. These standards typically include guidelines for soil management, pest and disease control, seed selection, animal welfare (if applicable), and restrictions on the use of synthetic chemicals, genetically modified organisms (GMOs), and irradiation.

Application:

• Producers interested in obtaining organic certification submit an application to a certifying agency or body. These agencies are typically accredited by government authorities and are responsible for ensuring that farmers and producers comply with organic standards.

Inspection:

• After receiving the application, the certifying agency conducts on-site inspections of the farm or production facility. Inspectors assess various aspects, including farming practices, record-keeping, storage, and transportation, to ensure compliance with organic standards.

Record Keeping:

• Organic producers are required to maintain detailed records of their farming practices. This includes information on seed sources, cultivation practices, pest management, and any inputs used on the farm. The record-keeping helps verify that organic standards have been consistently followed.

Certification Decision:

• Based on the inspection and review of records, the certifying agency makes a decision on whether to grant organic certification. If the farm or producer meets the required standards, they are issued an organic certification.

Labeling and Traceability:

• Once certified, the producer is allowed to use the organic label on their products. This label assures consumers that the product complies with organic standards. Additionally, the certification process includes traceability requirements to track the organic products from the farm to the market.

Annual Renewal:

• Organic certification is typically valid for a limited period, often one year. Producers must undergo annual inspections and renew their certification to ensure ongoing compliance with organic standards.

Certifying agencies play a crucial role in the organic certification process, and their accreditation is essential for ensuring the integrity of the organic label. Consumers can look for specific organic certification logos on product packaging to identify products that meet organic standards in their respective regions.

CHAPTER TWO
Advantages of Consuming Organic Food

Going for an organic diet can yield numerous possible advantages, although personal experiences and tastes may differ. Here are some frequently mentioned advantages of consuming organic food:

Reduced Exposure to Pesticides:

• Organic farming practices avoid the use of synthetic pesticides and herbicides. Choosing organic foods can help reduce exposure to these chemicals, which may be of particular concern for individuals aiming to minimize their intake of potentially harmful substances.

No Genetically Modified Organisms (GMOs):

• Organic standards prohibit the use of genetically modified organisms (GMOs) in the production of organic foods. For individuals concerned about the potential long-term health and environmental effects of GMOs, choosing organic can provide assurance of GMO-free products.

Nutrient Content:

• While research findings are mixed, some studies suggest that certain organic foods may have higher levels of certain nutrients and antioxidants compared to their conventionally grown counterparts. However, it's essential to note that the overall nutrient content can vary based on factors such as crop variety, soil quality, and growing conditions.

Environmental Impact:

• Organic farming practices often prioritize sustainability and environmental conservation. These practices may include crop rotation, reduced use of synthetic inputs, and promotion of biodiversity. Choosing organic can be seen as a way to support environmentally friendly and sustainable agriculture.

Animal Welfare:

• In the case of organic meat, dairy, and eggs, organic standards often include requirements for humane treatment of animals. This may involve providing access to outdoor areas, sufficient space, and restrictions on the use of antibiotics and growth hormones.

Soil Health:

• Organic farming methods focus on building and maintaining soil health through practices such as composting, cover cropping, and avoiding synthetic fertilizers. Healthy soil is essential for nutrient-rich crops and overall ecosystem sustainability.

Support for Sustainable Agriculture:

• By choosing organic products, consumers may be supporting farmers and producers who prioritize sustainable and environmentally responsible practices. This can contribute to the long-term health of agricultural ecosystems and communities.

Reduced Antibiotic Use:

• Organic standards typically restrict the routine use of antibiotics in animal farming. This can be beneficial in addressing concerns related to antibiotic resistance and promoting more responsible use of these medications in agriculture.

It's important to note that while these potential benefits are often associated with organic eating, individual dietary choices are multifaceted. People may choose organic foods for a combination of health, environmental, and ethical reasons. Additionally, maintaining a balanced and varied diet, whether organic or conventional, is key to overall well-being.

The Health Benefits of an Organic Diet

The health benefits of an organic diet have been a topic of research and discussion, though scientific consensus on some aspects is still evolving. Here are some potential health benefits associated with choosing an organic diet:

Reduced Pesticide Exposure:

• Organic farming avoids the use of synthetic pesticides and herbicides. Choosing organic foods can reduce exposure to residues from these chemicals, which has been a concern in conventional agriculture.

No Genetically Modified Organisms (GMOs):

• Organic standards prohibit the use of genetically modified organisms (GMOs). Some studies have raised questions about the long-term health effects of GMO consumption, and choosing organic can offer a GMO-free option for those with concerns.

Higher Antioxidant Content:

• Some studies suggest that certain organic fruits and vegetables may have higher levels of antioxidants and other beneficial compounds compared to their conventionally grown counterparts. Antioxidants play a role in neutralizing harmful free radicals in the body.

Nutrient Density:

• While findings are not consistent across all studies, some research indicates that organic crops may have higher nutrient density, including levels of certain vitamins and minerals. The nutrient content can be influenced by factors such as soil quality and farming practices.

Reduced Antibiotic and Hormone Exposure:

• Organic animal products often come from animals raised without the routine use of antibiotics and synthetic hormones. Limiting exposure to these substances in food may contribute to reducing the risk of antibiotic resistance and hormone-related health concerns.

Lower Presence of Heavy Metals:

• Some studies suggest that organic crops may have lower levels of certain heavy metals, such as cadmium. Reduced exposure to heavy metals in food is considered beneficial for human health.

Improved Heart Health:

• Limited research suggests that consuming organic dairy products may be associated with a more favorable fatty acid profile, potentially contributing to heart health. However, more research is needed to establish a clear link.

Possible Reduction in Allergenic Compounds:

• Some studies have explored the idea that organic crops may have lower levels of certain allergenic compounds, potentially benefiting individuals with sensitivities. However, research in this area is ongoing.

It's essential to note that while these potential benefits are suggested by some studies, the overall body of research is not entirely consistent, and more studies are needed to draw definitive conclusions. Additionally, the health benefits of an organic diet can vary depending on individual factors, including overall dietary choices, lifestyle, and health conditions. Maintaining a balanced and varied diet that includes a range of fruits, vegetables, and other nutrient-rich foods is key to overall health, whether the diet is organic or conventional.

CHAPTER THREE
Nutrient Content in Organic Food

The Nutritional Composition Of Organic Food Can Be Affected By Multiple Factors, Such As Soil Fertility, Agricultural Methods, And Plant Cultivars. Although Many Studies Indicate That Specific Organic Foods May Contain Modestly Elevated Quantities Of Certain Nutrients And Antioxidants, The Overall Distinctions Between Organic And Conventional Foods Are Not Consistently Evident. It Is Necessary To Acknowledge That The Nutritional Composition Of Any Product Can Fluctuate Due To Many Variables, And Individual Dietary Requirements Can Have A Significant Impact. Here Are Some Factors To

Consider Regarding The Nutritional Composition Of Organic Food:

1. **Soil Quality:**
    - Organic farming emphasizes soil health through practices like crop rotation, cover cropping, and the use of organic matter. Healthy soils contribute to better nutrient absorption by plants, potentially influencing the nutritional content of organic produce.

2. **Crop Variety:**
    - Different crop varieties may vary in their nutrient

content. The choice of organic versus conventional farming methods may not be the sole factor influencing nutrient levels; the specific crop variety and its inherent nutritional characteristics also play a role.

3. **Farming Practices:**

   - Organic farming avoids synthetic pesticides and fertilizers, relying on natural methods to maintain soil fertility. Some studies suggest that these practices may lead to differences in nutrient levels, but the results are not universally consistent across all crops.

4. **Antioxidants:**

   o Some research indicates that certain organic fruits and vegetables may have higher levels of antioxidants. Antioxidants are compounds that help neutralize free radicals in the body and are associated with various health benefits.

5. **Vitamin C and Polyphenols:**

   o Studies have suggested that certain organic fruits and vegetables, such as strawberries and apples, may contain higher levels of vitamin C and polyphenols, which have antioxidant properties.

6. **Nutrient Density:**

- The concept of nutrient density refers to the concentration of nutrients per unit of food. While some studies suggest that organic foods may have higher nutrient density, the evidence is not consistent across all food types.

It's important to approach the topic with a balanced perspective:

- **Overall Diet Matters:** The focus should be on maintaining a balanced and varied diet that includes a wide range of fruits, vegetables, whole grains, and other nutrient-rich foods, regardless of whether they are organic or conventional.

- **Individual Variability:** Nutritional needs can vary from person to person based on factors such as age, sex, health status, and lifestyle. A well-rounded diet is crucial for meeting individual nutritional requirements.

- **Research Continues:** The scientific understanding of the nutritional differences between organic and conventional foods is an ongoing area of research. As more studies are conducted, the evidence may evolve.

In summary, while some studies suggest potential differences in nutrient content between organic and conventional foods, the overall impact on human health is not fully established. Making informed choices based on personal preferences, values, and overall dietary patterns is key to a healthy and balanced diet.

Building Your Organic Kitchen

Creating an organic kitchen entails making deliberate decisions regarding the foods and goods you introduce into your house, prioritizing organic and eco-friendly alternatives. Below are some guidelines for constructing an organic kitchen:

• **Choose for Organic Produce:** Give priority to organic fruits and vegetables. Search for the USDA Organic or a comparable certification on the packaging. Opting to purchase local, seasonal products from farmers' markets or enrolling in a community-supported agriculture (CSA) program can also be a sustainable decision.

• Choose organic whole grains, cereals, and legumes. These commodities encompass organic rice, quinoa, oats, and lentils. Verify the presence of the organic certification on the packaging.

• **Opt for Organic Dairy and Eggs:** Select organic dairy products and eggs sourced from animals that are raised without the regular administration of antibiotics and synthetic hormones. Seek out the organic label on dairy products such as milk, cheese, and yogurt.

• **Select Organic Meat and Poultry:** If you consume meat, opt for organic alternatives. Organic meat is derived from animals that are reared on organic diet and are not regularly administered antibiotics or growth hormones. Seek out the organic certification on meat and poultry items.

• Investigate organic snacks and processed foods, as well as pantry essentials. Inspect the labels to ensure that the products have obtained organic certification and steer clear of those that contain synthetic ingredients, preservatives, and artificial colors.

• **Opt for Organic Beverages:** oPrioritize organic beverages such as organic coffee, tea, and juices. Several companies provide organic alternatives, which give a more sustainable and eco-friendly option.

• Opt for organic cooking oils, such as organic olive oil, coconut oil, or other varieties. Search for oils that have been extracted using the cold-press method and have undergone minimal processing.

• Acquire a Supply of Organic Herbs and Spices: o Utilize organic herbs and spices to enhance the taste of your meals. Seek organic alternatives to guarantee that these seasonings are devoid of artificial pesticides.

• Opt for local and seasonal organic produce whenever available. Local farmers' markets and CSA programs are wonderful sources for fresh, seasonal, and frequently organic foods.

• **Opt for Organic Cleaning Supplies**: Extend the principles of organic living to your cleaning routine by selecting ecologically conscious and organic cleaning solutions. These products frequently utilize components that are both natural and biodegradable.

• **Consider utilizing organic cookware and utensils:** Investigate the use of cookware and cooking utensils that are crafted from sustainable and organic resources. Materials such as bamboo, stainless steel, and cast iron are ecologically sustainable choices.

• **Decrease Food Waste**: Minimize food waste by engaging in conscious buying, employing appropriate storage techniques, and utilizing leftovers in innovative ways. This is in line with the environmental and resource-conscious concepts of organic living.

Keep in mind that constructing an organic kitchen is a step-by-step procedure, and it is OK to implement modifications gradually. Arrange in order of importance according to your financial resources, personal choices, and principles. Adopting tiny, sustainable decisions can have a positive impact on both your kitchen and your lifestyle, promoting better health.

CHAPTER FOUR

Organic Meal Planning

Organic meal planning involves creating well-balanced and nutritious meals while prioritizing organic, locally sourced, and sustainable ingredients. Here are some tips for effective organic meal planning:

1. **Start with a Weekly Plan:**
   - Plan your meals for the week ahead. Consider your schedule, and think about which days you'll have more time to cook and when you may need quick and easy options.

2. **Create a Shopping List:**

- Based on your meal plan, make a shopping list of the organic ingredients you need. Organize the list by categories (produce, dairy, grains, etc.) to make your shopping trip more efficient.

3. **Prioritize Seasonal and Local Produce:**

   - Include seasonal and local organic produce in your meal plan. Seasonal fruits and vegetables are often fresher, more flavorful, and may be more affordable. Visit farmers' markets or join a community-supported agriculture (CSA) program for local, organic options.

4. **Incorporate a Variety of Whole Foods:**

   o Build your meals around a variety of whole foods, including organic grains, legumes, fruits, vegetables, nuts, and seeds. This ensures a diverse range of nutrients in your diet.

5. **Choose Organic Protein Sources:**

   o Include organic sources of protein in your meals. This could be organic meat, poultry, fish, eggs, tofu, tempeh, or legumes. Aim for a balance of plant-based and animal-based proteins.

6. **Plan for Leftovers:**

    o Cook larger batches and plan for leftovers to save time on busy days. This reduces the need for frequent cooking and helps minimize food waste.

7. **Experiment with Meatless Meals:**

    o Include meatless meals in your plan, such as vegetarian or vegan options. Plant-based meals can be rich in nutrients and environmentally friendly.

8. **Incorporate Whole Grains:**

   o Choose organic whole grains like brown rice, quinoa, oats, and whole wheat. These grains provide fiber and essential nutrients.

9. **Use Organic Herbs and Spices:**

   o Enhance the flavor of your meals with organic herbs and spices. This adds variety to your dishes without relying on excessive salt or processed seasonings.

10. **Minimize Processed Foods:**

o Reduce the inclusion of processed and packaged foods in your meal plan. Opt for whole, minimally processed options to maximize nutritional value.

11. **Plan for Snacks:**

o Include organic snacks in your meal plan to help curb hunger between meals. Options can include fresh fruits, raw nuts, yogurt, or cut-up vegetables with hummus.

12. **Stay Flexible:**

o Be flexible and open to adjustments. Life can be unpredictable, and sometimes plans change. Having a flexible approach allows you to adapt your meals as needed.

13. **Practice Sustainable Cooking:**

   o Practice sustainable cooking by using energy-efficient appliances, minimizing food waste, and choosing eco-friendly kitchen practices.

Remember to enjoy the process of cooking and experimenting with different flavors and ingredients. Organic meal planning not only contributes to your health but also supports sustainable and environmentally conscious practices.

Organic Products Suitable For All Types of Lifestyles.

Embracing an organic lifestyle can be customized to suit different preferences, nutritional preferences, and ways of living. Regardless of whether you follow a vegetarian, vegan, omnivorous, or have specific dietary requirements, you can incorporate organic principles into your way of life. Here are methods to adopt organic choices that are appropriate for various lifestyles:

1. Vegetarian and Vegan Lifestyles: Prioritize the consumption of plant-based organic foods, including fruits, vegetables, legumes, nuts, seeds, and whole grains.

• Opt for organic plant-based protein sources such as tofu, tempeh, and organic beans.

Discover a range of organic plant-based milk substitutes, such as organic soy milk, almond milk, or oat milk.

2. Omnivorous Lifestyles: Choose organic meats, poultry, and fish as sources of animal-based protein.

• Include organic dairy products, eggs, and other animal products sourced from producers that adhere to organic farming methods.

Strive for a harmonious combination of organic plant-based and animal-based foods to provide a varied intake of nutrients.

3. Maintaining a Healthy Lifestyle: Make organic whole foods, such as fruits, vegetables, whole grains, and lean proteins, a top priority.

• Reduce the use of processed and packaged foods, opting for organic options whenever possible.

Integrate natural herbs and spices to increase taste without depending on excessive salt or processed flavors.

4. For athletic and fitness lifestyles, it is recommended to incorporate organic sources of energy, such as organic fruits, nuts, and whole grains, into your pre-workout snacks.

Choose organic protein sources to aid in muscle rehabilitation, such as organic meat, chicken, fish, eggs, and plant-based alternatives like organic tofu or tempeh.

5. For individuals with busy and active lifestyles, it is advisable to go for handy organic snacks that can be easily consumed while on the move. Examples of such snacks are organic trail mix, fresh fruits, or organic granola bars.

• Consider seeking pre-cut organic vegetables or pre-washed organic salad mixtures as a time-saving measure for dinner preparation.

6. Promoting Family and Kid-Friendly Lifestyles: early introduction of organic fruits and vegetables to children, with a focus on highlighting their significance for maintaining good health.

• Include organic whole grains, dairy products, and lean proteins in your family's meals.

• Involve youngsters in the practice of organic gardening or in the activity of shopping for organic produce to provide an enjoyable and informative experience.

7. Embracing Sustainable and Eco-Friendly Lifestyles: Opt for organic products that come in environmentally-friendly packaging, or contemplate purchasing items in bulk to minimize waste.

• Support local farmers and producers by buying organic, locally sourced food.

• To reduce food waste, one should employ strategies such as meal planning, innovative use of leftovers, and composting of organic waste.

8. Special Dietary Needs: Investigate organic alternatives that cater to special dietary requirements, such as gluten-free, lactose-free, or nut-free organic options.

Verify the presence of organic certification on specialist items in order to guarantee that they adhere to certain dietary needs.

To successfully embrace an organic lifestyle, it is crucial to select options that are in harmony with your principles, personal preferences, and health objectives. This strategy is versatile and can be customized to suit different lifestyles, thereby making organic choices available to all individuals.

Recipes for an Organic Lifestyle

Adopting an organic lifestyle often involves incorporating whole, minimally processed ingredients into your meals. Here are a few organic recipes that emphasize fresh, organic produce and sustainable ingredients:

1. **Quinoa Salad with Roasted Vegetables:**

Ingredients:

- 1 cup quinoa (organic)
- Assorted organic vegetables (e.g., bell peppers, cherry tomatoes, zucchini, red onion)
- Olive oil (organic)
- Balsamic vinegar (organic)
- Fresh basil (organic), chopped

- Salt and pepper to taste

Instructions:

A. Cook quinoa according to package instructions.

B. Chop vegetables and toss with olive oil, salt, and pepper. Roast in the oven until tender.

C. Mix cooked quinoa and roasted vegetables. Drizzle with balsamic vinegar, and sprinkle with fresh basil.

2. Organic Chickpea and Vegetable Stir-Fry:

Ingredients:

- 1 can organic chickpeas, drained and rinsed

- Mixed organic vegetables (e.g., broccoli, bell peppers, snap peas, carrots)
- Organic tofu, cubed
- Organic soy sauce
- Sesame oil (organic)
- Garlic and ginger, minced
- Brown rice (organic)

Instructions:

A. Stir-fry tofu until golden in sesame oil. Add garlic and ginger.

B. Add mixed vegetables and chickpeas. Stir-fry until vegetables are tender yet crisp.

C. Pour soy sauce over the stir-fry and toss until well coated. Serve over cooked brown rice.

3. **Organic Berry Smoothie Bowl:**

Ingredients:

- Organic mixed berries (strawberries, blueberries, raspberries)
- Organic banana, sliced
- Organic Greek yogurt
- Organic granola
- Chia seeds (organic)
- Honey (organic), optional

Instructions:

A. Blend mixed berries and banana until smooth.
B. Pour the smoothie into a bowl and top with Greek yogurt, granola, chia seeds, and sliced berries.

C. Drizzle with honey if desired.

4. Spaghetti with Organic Tomato Sauce and Roasted Garlic:

Ingredients:

- Whole-grain or organic spaghetti
- Organic tomato sauce
- Organic cherry tomatoes, halved
- Organic garlic cloves
- Fresh basil (organic), chopped
- Olive oil (organic)
- Salt and pepper to taste
- Grated Parmesan cheese (organic), optional

Instructions:

> A. Roast garlic cloves in olive oil until golden.
>
> B. Cook spaghetti according to package instructions.
>
> C. Mix cooked spaghetti with tomato sauce, roasted garlic, cherry tomatoes, and fresh basil. Season with salt and pepper.
>
> D. Serve with a sprinkle of grated Parmesan cheese if desired.

5. Organic Green Salad with Lemon Tahini Dressing:

Ingredients:

- Mixed organic salad greens (e.g., kale, spinach, arugula)

- Cherry tomatoes, halved
- Cucumber, sliced
- Avocado, diced
- Pumpkin seeds (organic)
- Dressing: Tahini (organic), lemon juice, olive oil, salt, and pepper

Instructions:

A. Toss mixed greens, cherry tomatoes, cucumber, and avocado in a large bowl.

B. In a separate bowl, whisk together tahini, lemon juice, olive oil, salt, and pepper for the dressing.

C. Drizzle the dressing over the salad and sprinkle with pumpkin seeds.

Feel free to customize these recipes based on your taste preferences and seasonal availability of organic produce. Enjoy your journey towards a delicious and sustainable organic lifestyle!

Conclusion

Embracing an organic lifestyle entails making conscientious decisions regarding the food we consume, the goods we utilize, and the influence we exert on the environment. By giving priority to organic choices, individuals can enhance their overall health, promote sustainable agricultural methods, and diminish their impact on the environment.

• When it comes to food, opting for organic means choosing produce that has been grown without the use of artificial pesticides, herbicides, and genetically modified organisms. It entails providing assistance to farmers who give priority to soil health, biodiversity, and the ethical treatment of animals. Although the nutritional disparities between organic and conventional foods may differ, the overarching focus on natural, sustainable methods is in line with a comprehensive approach to health.

• Having knowledge about labels and certifications enables consumers to make well-informed decisions when selecting products, whether they choose USDA Organic, Non-GMO Project Verified, Fair Trade, or any other certified options. These labels demonstrate a dedication to particular criteria, such as ecological sustainability, equitable labor practices, or the exclusion of genetically modified ingredients.

• Constructing an organic kitchen entails choosing organic ingredients and integrating environmentally friendly activities. Meal planning using organic foods, selecting sustainably sourced items, and reducing food waste are essential components of an organic kitchen.

• Recipes tailored for an organic lifestyle highlight the wide range and delectability of organic ingredients. These dishes prioritize the use of fresh, organic fruit and whole, minimally processed meals. Whether you're eating a quinoa salad with roasted veggies, an organic chickpea and vegetable stir-fry, or a refreshing berry smoothie bowl, the focus is on using high-quality ingredients.

To summarize, adopting an organic lifestyle is a comprehensive process that goes beyond personal decisions. It includes a dedication to individual welfare, ecological sustainability, and moral issues. Through deliberate choices in our everyday activities, we have the ability to actively participate in creating a healthier and more sustainable planet, both for ourselves and for future generations.

THE END